I0428558

# The Ultimate Guide to PAIN MANAGEMENT

## *How to Achieve Pain Relief & Live Pain Free for Life*

*MIA SOLEIL*

© **Copyright 2014 by Joy Publishing & Marketing Corporation - All rights reserved.**

This document is geared towards providing helpful and reliable information in regards to the topic and issue covered. The publication is sold with the idea that the publisher is not required to render accounting, officially permitted, or otherwise, qualified services. If advice is necessary, legal or professional, a practiced individual in the profession should be ordered.

- From a Declaration of Principles which was accepted and approved equally by a Committee of the American Bar Association and a Committee of Publishers and Associations.

In no way is it legal to reproduce, duplicate, or transmit any part of this document in either electronic means or in printed format. Recording of this publication is strictly prohibited and any storage of this document is not allowed unless with written permission from the publisher. All rights reserved.

The information provided herein is stated to be truthful and consistent, in that any liability, in terms of inattention or otherwise, by any usage or abuse of any policies, processes, or directions contained within is the solitary and utter responsibility of the recipient reader. Under no circumstances will any legal responsibility or blame be held against the publisher for any reparation, damages, or monetary loss due to the information herein, either directly or indirectly.

Respective authors own all copyrights not held by the publisher.

The information herein is offered for informational purposes solely, and is universal as so. The presentation of the information is without contract or any type of guarantee assurance.

The trademarks that are used are without any consent, and the publication of the trademark is without permission or backing by the trademark owner. All trademarks and brands within this book are for clarifying purposes only and are the owned by the owners themselves, not affiliated with this document

.

# Table of Contents

# Introduction

I want to thank you and congratulate you for purchasing this book!

This book contains proven steps and strategies on how to recognize and differentiate types of pain and their causes. The main insight this book will provide, the one that we're all craving for, is how to achieve pain relief. The goal was to create a book rich in practical techniques and strategies for achieving the relief from pain that we all so desperately desire. Once we are able to bring our bodies into a pain free reality, the challenge is to prevent relapse. We'll conclude with strategies for promoting this lasting change.

I personally have struggled with chronic pain in the forms of lower back and neck pain, and headaches. From Elementary to Secondary school, I had a headache almost every day. I actually didn't know what it was like to NOT have a headache. I frequently took pain relieving medicines like Tylenol and Advil to help cope with the daily pain. In the end, it was actually my sinuses that were contributing to the problem all along. Once I was able to deal with the root of the problem, rather than the symptoms, I saw a drastic turn around.

I also had a serious accident that was so powerful, I knocked down a lamp post! I didn't feel the effects of this car accident till about six years later. The accident and progression of poor posture and stress caused my chronic neck pain to rear its ugly head. That led to a sloughs of chiropractor and massage therapy appointments over the next several years.

In December 2010, I gave birth to my daughter. I was originally very scared of the anticipated pain of childbirth. I couldn't imagine how it would all physically take place. Through a series of events and an adjustment of my thinking, which I'll save for another book, I was able to be at peace with labor. I successfully gave birth naturally, in my own home, without any form of pain medication. Keep in mind: this is coming from the same person that would take Tylenol for a simple headache because I was such a wimp when it came to dealing with pain.

Our lives should not be crippled because of pain. We shouldn't have to settle for less than awesome because of the debilitating effects of chronic pain in our daily lives. We shouldn't have to sit on the sidelines because we're in too much pain to play the game. Everyone that has been on this journey knows the cost of trying to achieve a pain free life – it is a costly one. It stops here! My hope for you is that this is the last price to be paid on your chronic pain.

I sincerely thank you for purchasing this book. I truly hope you enjoy it! I hope you are able to gain insight, encouragement and strategies to apply to your life to receive the joy and peace you deserve.

Please take some time to stop by and LIKE our Facebook page:

https://www.facebook.com/joypublishing

With gratitude,

*Mia Soleil*

# Chapter 1

# Pain and the Body

When you cut yourself, blood oozes out and there's a sharp pain that follows. If you have a migraine, you feel a chronic throbbing pain in your head. If you are burnt, pain is intensely unbearable. These are different scenarios where a person undergoes a painful experience. Pain in varying degrees of intensity and frequency is identified. The definition of pain, however, is out of the question.

## What is Pain?

Pain is a complex stimulus. There is no exact definition because it is an entirely subjective sensation. It is the foremost reason why people seek medical attention. Pain tells you that something is wrong or damaged. The International Association for the Study of Pain defines it as "an unpleasant sensory and emotional experience associated with actual or potential tissue damage or described in terms of such damage".

In actual context, pain is not always associated with physiological processes. Medical attention can identify and treat physical pain, but there's also another kind of pain which is really hard if not impossible to treat through medical means...emotional pain. So what is pain? Pain, to put it simply, is far more than neural transmission and sensory transduction. It is a complex mixture of emotion, sensation, culture, experience and spirit.

## How Does the Body React to Pain?

Pain perception or nociception is the process where a painful stimulus is signaled and relayed to the central nervous system from the point of origin. It is entirely different when compared to normal stimuli like touch, ordinary pressure and temperature. When the stimulus is non-painful, normal somatic receptors are the first to act. If it is a painful stimulation, nociceptors are the first to fire up.

This process includes several steps:

1. *Point of origin or contact with stimulus* - the point of origin can be mechanical such as cuts, pressures, abrasions and pressure. It can also be chemically inflicted like burns.

2. *Reception* - It is a process where the nerve ending senses the stimulus.

3. *Transmission* - When nerve endings sense the stimulus, they transmit the signal to the central nervous system through a series of neurons.

4. *Perception* - This is where the brain receives the signal for further processing and action.

When you cut your hand, there are several factors that contribute to your perception of pain. First is the mechanical stimulation of the sharp object that cut you. Your cells are damaged and they release potassium. This is why you feel the intense sharp pain at the moment of injury. Then Prostaglandins, histamines and bradykinins from the immune cells invade the area during inflammation. This is the stage where your body is protecting you from the foreign stimulus. You will experience a longer dull ache or numbing feeling along the affected area.

Nociceptor neurons travel in peripheral sensory nerves. The signals are relayed from the free nerve endings at the layer of the skin. These signals are sent to the spinal cord through the dorsal roots. They synapse on the neurons within the spinal cord segment and also two or three segments below and above the point of entry. This is basically the reason why it is sometimes difficult to locate the location of the pain in the body especially when the damage is internal.

Secondary neurons then transmit the signal upward through the spinothalamic tract. The signal travels from the spinothalamic tract to the medulla (brain's system) and ends in the thalamus, which is the central relaying center of the brain. Some neurons also send signal to the medulla's reticular receptors which control the physical behavior.

Once the signal is processed in the brain, some signals will pass through the motor cortex, to the spinal cord then down to the motor nerves. These impulses cause muscle contractions that make you move your hand away from the object.

**What are the Types of Pain?**

There are different types of pain. Neuroscientists and physicians classify pain in three ways:

1. *Acute Pain* - This is a type of pain which is inflicted to the body. An injury to the body like a cut or burn causes an acute pain in the affected area. It warns of potential damage and compels action from the brain. It can develop slowly or quickly. Depending on the type of injury and the intensity of the damage, pain can last up to a few minutes to a year. When the wound starts to heal however, acute pain goes away.

2. *Chronic Pain* - It is a persistent kind of pain. It does not require your body to respond unlike acute pain. Chronic pain still persists even when the trauma has been healed. It lasts longer than six months. An example of a chronic pain is a migraine.

3. *Cancer/Malignant Pain* - This is a kind of pain associated with tumors. It is somehow associated with chronic pain; however, cancer pain is more painful and affects a wider area. This is because tumors invade healthy cells thus, affecting nearby blood vessels and nerves.

# Chapter 2

# Pain Management in Medical Context

When a person goes to a hospital for pain treatment, physicians treat it in numerous possible ways. Pain management consists of medication such as taking an aspirin or ibuprofen as a pain reliever; surgery, which is common to more serious injuries like gunshots, burns, and organ failures; alternative procedures like hypnosis, massage therapy and acupuncture; or a combination of these approaches.

The type of medication prescribed depends on the source of pain, side effects of the medication, health status of the person and the level of discomfort experienced by the afflicted.

1.  **Medication**: There are different types of medication given to a patient at a certain time and scenario.

    *   *Non-Opioid Analgesics* - This includes aspirin, ibuprofen, acetaminophen and naproxen. They are used as pain relievers and they act on the site of pain directly. When the tissue is damaged, an enzyme is released and local pain or the pain on the affected area is produced. This type of medication prevents the onset of these enzymes, soothes the pain and reduces inflammation. This type of analgesics, however, can have adverse effects on the kidneys and liver and causes internal bleeding and gastrointestinal discomfort when usage is prolonged.

    *   *Opioid Analgesics* - This medication is applied to higher and more intense levels of pain. They act on the synaptic neurons and

activate downward pathways of signals. They target various parts in the central nervous system by binding to Opioid receptors. This includes morphine, codeine, meripidine, fentanyl, propoxyphine, and oxycodone. The side effect can be addictive and over dosage is likely to occur at different times.

- *Adjuvant Analgesics* - These are also pain relievers but they are used to treat other conditions. They act against neuropathic pain or the pain caused by damage to the central nervous system. This includes tricyclic anti-depressants, anti-epileptic drugs and anesthetics.

2. **Surgery**: Surgery is always the last resort. When all the pain relievers no longer alleviate pain, surgery must be done to sever pain pathways. Two types of surgery include Rhizotomy, which destroys portions of the peripheral nerves; and Achordotomy, which destroys ascending tracts to the spinal cord preventing the pain signal receptors in reaching the medulla or the brain system.

3. **Alternative Therapy**: This does not involve drugs or surgery. It includes chiropracty (manipulates joints to relieve nerve pressures), massage, hot compress, acupuncture (stimulates nerves and release endorphins) and mental control such as hypnosis which rely on the brain to alleviate pain.

# Chapter 3

# How does pain affect your Life?

Pain can affect your life in numerous ways. If you are a professional and have to go to work, if you experience pain, your work is affected. You will not be able to concentrate on finishing your tasks if something is wrong with you. If you are sick, you have to be absent for treatment or rest. Either way, your work is still affected. If you are a parent, how can you take care of your kids if you are hurt? Pain, is of course a natural stimulus that should not be taken for granted. The more you ignore the pain, the worse your situation may become.

If pain is chronic, it has a detrimental effect on the everyday life of the person. It affects the patient's ability to perform natural functions and responsibilities. Physical activities are limited. Chronic pain is also associated with depression, anxiety, sleep disturbances and panic attacks. Chronic pain also impedes mobility or flexibility of the patient as it may result to difficulty in walking or carrying things, poor personal hygiene, and loss of social contacts with family and friends, and constipation and incontinence.

Chronic pain affects you physically and psychologically. It limits what you can do. It interferes with your ability to work, play with your children or grandchildren; it also diminishes your ability to take care of your own self. When these happen, pain causes you to feel useless and incompetent, making you succumb to a depressed state. People with chronic pain often experience irritability, anger, depression, and difficulty in concentrating. It becomes as debilitating as the pain itself.

Pain changes a person's personality. Coping with chronic pain, on the other hand, calls for a great deal of change and introspection from the person itself. It pressures the person while he is trying to

9

hide the pain and forces himself to cover the handicap by a sense of forged well-being to be functional.

- The Pain Haze - Chronic pain is unpredictable. It is sometimes mild and other times, it is unbearable. When a person is in pain, his perception about things is obscured and his responses are slow. This is the stage where a person's personality does not reflect on the outside.

- Mental Health Condition - Pain causes sleeplessness and mood swings. Chronic pain leads to painful depressions and helplessness which, in turn leads to suicidal tendencies, anxiety and panic disorders.

- Perception - People who are in painful situations are always misunderstood. Oftentimes, their real perception and intentions are not reflected on the outside. Their ways of coping with pain is essentially vital to how people view them. Their view of life is also affected. Those who suffer from serious illnesses perceive life as something they have to live to the fullest as their time is already counted and the likes. Some also become hopeless and afraid of the things to come.

# Chapter 4

# Natural Pain Relievers

There are many circumstances where prescribed medications just won't work. There are also times when your body does not respond positively to treatments. If you have allergic reactions to certain medications, especially pain relievers and anesthetics, it is best that you use natural alternatives instead for pain treatment. Nature is still the best healer. There are wonderful herbs out there that contain extracts effective in reducing inflammation and infection. Here are a few of them:

1.  *Capsaicin*: This is an active component found in chili pepper. It temporarily desensitizes C fibers which are the pain-prone nerve receptors. If applied on the injured area, Capsaicin diminishes soreness for three to five weeks until the nerves regain sensation. It has already been proven effective and is now commercially sold and used worldwide. It has been reported that forty percent of arthritis patients experienced fifty percent pain reduction after one month of using capsaicin cream.

2.  *Inflathera and Zyflamend*: These two components are both present in ginger, turmeric and holy basil which are all anti-inflammatory agents. Turmeric, which is also an ingredient used primarily in delicious curry meals, is one of the best natural pain relievers. New research suggests that turmeric contains curcumin, which eases inflammatory conditions like rheumatoid arthritis and psoriasis. It also has anti-cancer properties. Furthermore, turmeric also helps in blood circulation and prevents blood clotting. Curcumin lowers the amount of enzymes released by the damaged cells and reduces the pain in the body. It is best used to treat, bruises, joint inflammation, skin and digestive issues. Ginger on the other hand, has been used to relieve pain since thousands of years ago by the Chinese

people. It relieves nausea, arthritis, headaches, menstrual cramps, muscle soreness and blood circulation issues.

3. *Valerian Root*: Valerian root is also called nature's tranquilizers. It regulates the central nervous system thereby relieving insomnia, tension, irritability or mood swings, anxiety and stress. A cup of Valerian aids in pain relief by reducing sensitivity of the nerves.

4. *Salicin*: This is a component commonly found in aspirins. It is also naturally found in white willow barks. This traditional pain reliever is used to treat painful joint inflammation. White willow bark effects are slower than the commercial aspirin but it is much longer. Contrary to aspirin, white willow bark does not upset the stomach and won't damage gastro-intestinal lining. It was also discovered that white willow bark reduces the severity of migraine attacks.

5. *Arnica*: Arnica is a component found active in a European flower. Although the healing mechanism remains unknown, it does contain anti-inflammatory properties. This is best applied to relieve acute injury or post-surgery swelling. Taking oral homeopathic arnica after a surgery reduces painful swelling.

6. *Herbal and Fish Oil*: Herbal or Tonic oil such as peppermint, camphor, eucalyptus, fennel and wintergreen can be used to treat migraine or normal headaches. They can be applied topically on the affected area and their menthol or cooling properties reduce pain and inflammation. Digested fish oils on the other hand, when broken down, become prostaglandin, which are powerful agents that reduce inflammation. In one study, about 40 percent of patients suffering from rheumatic arthritis who have taken cod-liver oil for a month were able to cut their NSAIDS intake by a third. Two-thirds of people who experience neck and back pains were able to stop using

NSAIDS altogether after 10 weeks of taking cod-liver fish oil.

7. *Methysulfonyl-Methane (MSM)*: This is an active component of sulfur and it prevents joint and cartilage degeneration. In an experiment conducted by the University of California in San Diego, scientists reported that people with osteoarthritis who took MSM have experienced twenty-five percent less pain and are thirty percent more physically active than their counterparts who didn't.

8. *Apple Cider Vinegar*: This contains alkaline forming properties necessary for the body. One tablespoon of apple cider vinegar relieves the person of the painful spasms caused by heart burn. It also contains over-all alkalizing effects which the body desperately needs during this modern era of acid-forming diets.

9. *Bromelain*: An active component of pineapple, it is known to relieve bloated tummy and heaviness. It also improves blood circulation, preventing blood clots, inhibits inflammation, and stops muscle and menstrual cramps. It is recommended to those who suffer from arthritis.

10. *Garlic*: In the olden times, garlic was the most popular pain reliever. It is a home remedy for tooth-ache and other skin problems such as psoriasis and acne. Garlic contains anti-fungal and anti-inflammatory properties that are best for pain treatment and healing.

11. *Oats*: Oats are believed to have powerful effects in the reduction of menstrual cramps. It also relives endometriosis. They contain magnesium and are the best sources of dietary zinc necessary for women who always suffer from painful menstrual periods.

12. *Grapes*: An Ohio University research study shows that 1 cup of grapes when eaten on a daily basis reduces the risks and frequency of suffering from back pains. They are said to contain nutrients that aid in the blood circulation, thus alleviating pain.

13. *Blueberries*: They contain anti-oxidants which kill free radicals that enflame the digestive lining, thereby reducing severity of gastrointestinal pain.

In addition to this long list of natural pain relievers, are several practitioners that you may already familiar with. Some of these services complement each other. Often chronic pain is a compounded and complex issue. It's like an onion with several layers. It is not uncommon to partner several of these services together. They all support each other in helping peel away the layers.

1. *Chiropracty*: Chiropractors focus on the neuromusculoskeletal system and the connection the spine has with the rest of the body. They believe that misalignment or subluxations can even occur during the process of birth. When our body is out of alignment, chronic conditions and pain is created in the body. The chiropractor physically manipulates the joints to relieve nerve pressure and facilitate healing. Often, the muscles around the spine need to be taught to have a "new memory" so that pain relief can be maintained.

2. *Massage Therapy*: massage therapy can often go hand in hand with other forms of physical therapy. The practice focuses on manipulating the muscles and connective tissues in the body through a variety of techniques. The American Heritage dictionary says "massage is the rubbing or kneading of parts of the body to aid circulation or relax the muscles." Chronic pain can be alleviated when the muscles are relaxed and able to function as they were designed. Massage therapy can come in many forms such

as deep tissue massage, Swedish massage, Shiatsu and many more.

3. *Chinese Medicine*: Chinese medicine is based on 5000 years of tradition. It usually encompasses herbal medicine, acupuncture, massage, exercise and diet.

4. *Acupuncture/Acupressure*: stimulates nerves and release endorphins based on the different pressure points in the body. Acupuncture places needles into the skin along specific meridians and acupuncture points. Acupressure uses fingers, hands or other instruments instead of needles.

5. *Physiotherapy*: it is not uncommon to use physiotherapy after some form of serious accident that has disabled the body in some way. Usually after an accident, the body has a limited range of motion or is not able to perform the way it was intended. Physiotherapy treats the body's disease, injury or deformity by the means of physical techniques rather than drugs or surgery. These techniques include massage, stretching, exercise and heat treatment.

6. *Naturopathy*: According to the Canadian Association of Naturopathic Doctors, "naturopathic medicine is a distinct primary health care system that blends modern scientific knowledge with traditional and natural forms of medicine. The naturopathic philosophy is to stimulate the healing power of the body and treat the underlying cause of disease. Symptoms of disease are seen as warning signals of improper functioning of the body, and unfavorable lifestyle habits. In addition to diet and lifestyle changes, natural therapies including botanical medicine, clinical nutrition, hydrotherapy, homeopathy, naturopathic manipulation and traditional Chinese medicine/acupuncture, may also be used during treatments."

7. *Aromatherapy*: there is a powerful connection between the olfactory system and the aroma of essential oils. Different herbs have different healing properties that are capable of treating a variety of chronic conditions. Aromatherapy can be used in several ways from lighting a candle, applying to pressure points, spritzing on a pillow or adding to a hot bath. For example, basil is used for migraines while lavender is used as an anti-inflammatory.

8. *Hypnotherapy*: Hypnotherapy is a skilled verbal communication which helps direct a client's imagination in such a way as to bring about intended alterations in sensations, perceptions, feelings, thoughts and behavior (National Hypnotherapy Society). Hypnotherapy has been known to be successfully used during childbirth to help women manage pain during labor. Hypnotherapy can be self-taught or implemented from a trained therapist.

9. *Yoga*: yoga or simple stretching are simple practices that should be applied to everyday life to reduce the tension of stress and keep the muscles in proper working order. There are specific stretches that can focus on problem areas such as the neck or lower back. These stretches can be assigned from a personal trainer, massage therapist or physiotherapist. Yoga can be enjoyed at home or in a studio with several other participants. There are many forms of yoga ranging from hatha yoga to hot yoga. The focus in yoga is on breath control, meditation, stretching and balance. Not all forms of yoga are spiritual with chants and mantras if you don't feel comfortable with that form of practice.

# Chapter 5

# What aggravates pain?

Several studies and researches have been conducted, but until now, researchers are still clueless as to the things that aggravate pain. It was discovered, however, that the things which can alleviate pain are also the same things that can aggravate it. Furthermore, according to their studies, people generally do not know what exactly are the things or factors that can alleviate or aggravate their pain. Here are several factors:

1. *Activity*: Activity can aggravate the pain and worsen the situation. For example, a person who sprained his ankle is not allowed to move freely without a cane or support. If he uses his feet without support, the sprained ankle will have to carry the full weight thus, applying pressure on the injured ankle will make it worse and walking will be more painful. Changing positions can also aggravate pain because it adds pressure and force on the injured area.

2. *Foods and Oral Activities*: Eating is sometimes helpful, but oftentimes, it aggravates pain as well. When the person is sick, it is best to give him soft foods like mashed potatoes or porridge. In some situations however, even soft foods are still painful. Just the act of opening the mouth is already painful in some situations. Chewing is not advisable for tooth aches and during post dental surgeries. Intake of acidic foods and liquids is also prohibited, especially in the case of ulcer and canker sores. Kissing or talking is equally painful when the lip is busted or when there's a wound in the mouth. Furthermore, certain foods can cause adverse reactions in the body. For example, acidic type foods can exasperate arthritis symptoms. Gluten and milk products are known to elevate symptoms in the body causing inflammation.

3. *Inactivity*: As much as activity aggravates pain, inactivity can also aggravate it. Inactivity causes blood circulation to be stagnant and it produces pain. It produces a numbing pain when you sit for long period of time. If you are hospitalized and your position is unchanged for several days, you will develop bed sores and it's painful.

4. *Stress*: Stress also is a contributing factor that aggravates pain. Stress is known to be the "silent killer." When the body perceives a threat, it enters into a "fight or flight" response. When we are prepared to "fight", the adrenaline in our body increases and the cortisol hormone rises. This is normal and usually drops off when the stress is dealt with. However, if a person is in constant stress and has an overexposure to cortisol in the body, their health is quick to deteriorate and the body's healing process is ruptured. Sleeplessness also impedes the immune system from working properly thus, inflammation and swelling becomes worse. A fresh wound can also start to bleed and may reopen if a person is emotionally unstable, angry, or depressed.

5. *Medical Treatment*: As much as medical treatment can alleviate and relieve pain altogether, it can also make it worse. There are medications which produce harmful and painful side effects to the person being treated. For example, aspirins; they are indeed pain relievers and very powerful at that, however, when taken on a daily basis, it destroys gastrointestinal lining causing painful spasms and acute pain in the stomach. Chemotherapy is also another factor which aggravates pain, as well as surgery.

6. *Touch/Applications*: In severe physical injuries, pressure is needed to stop the bleeding. There are times however, when touching the injured area is not very advisable. This is true with those injured in motor or vehicular accidents. One wrong touch on the affected area can kill the person or worsen the injury. There may be broken bones which are better left untouched and without pressure. Similarly, if the

affected area is already infected and swelling is really severe, touching it becomes unbearably painful. This is the case of burn victims. The skin or the flesh is open and touching it is ultimately the most painful thing that they will hope never to experience. Antiseptic or cleaning their wound will make them cry in pain that is incomparable to anything else.

7. *Temperature* - Temperature can also aggravate the pain. This is most often the case for older people. Arthritis and other joint problems are at their most painful during the winter season. Bone cancer patients are most susceptible to severe pain during the cold season. Skin problems on the other hand, are most painful during the hot season or summer when the skin becomes dry. This is most particularly true when perspiration seeps into the wound.

8. *Posture* - Poor posture can also exasperate the pain, especially for people who suffer back and neck pain. Slouching, sitting too long, standing with one hip jutting out, twisting the body, improper lifting, crossing legs, or caring a backpack on one shoulder are many of the ways that our bodies can be thrown out of alignment. It is important to get up and stretch when sitting in a chair or car for too long. Every couple hours is recommended. When watching television, face the screen head on rather than twisting your body to view the screen. Practice sitting up right when at the computer or using electronic devises. It is best to not keep your head in the down position for too long. Movement is the key to keeping muscles loose in the body.

9. *Toxins* - environmental toxins can contribute to inflammation in the body and elevate the chronic pain. Toxins can include air quality, heavy metals in food or materials, pesticides, chemical fertilizers, antibiotics and hormones in food products, genetically modified foods, plastic containers, and nitrates in deli meats, artificial coloring/flavors/sweeteners, and chemical detergents. The

list is endless. Eliminating or reducing these toxins in your environment is crucial. People even go another step further and partake in routine detoxes and cleanses to rid the body of these harmful toxins.

# Chapter 6

# How to Prevent Relapses

A relapse is that part of the recovery process when a person may tend to go back to his ineffective pain management ways, giving rise to yet another round of pain. It is a common symptom that may be brought about by drug or medical dependency inherent to two-thirds of the patients who have experienced chronic pain despite their intention not to do so. Having said that, relapse is more properly defined as a progressive series of events that takes someone away from stable recovery to a state of becoming dysfunctional in their current recovery.

There are several ways on how people who have recovered can prevent painful relapses:

1.  *Do Not Overwork Yourself*: It is natural that the body will feel so much better and stronger after a series of treatments. In chronic pain, it is logical that people with this condition know what things trigger their physical pain the most. To prevent the pain in coming back again and persisting for longer periods of time, the person should not overwork himself. He should still rest until completely recovered. Only then can he or she be able to sustain full recovery.

2.  *Stay Rested and Have a Good Sleep*: Nothing is better than a good night's sleep to detoxify and cleanse the body. Sleep helps in repairing tissues and corroded cells. If you sleep at night and you are well-rested, your body will be able to recuperate faster.

3.  *Relapse Education*: This is the most vital stage in relapse prevention. The relapser needs to be educated. He needs to understand that what he is going through is a normal stage in the process of recovery and that there is something he

can do to overcome it. The person needs to be sober from drugs or any medication for him to understand it.

4. *Live a Balanced Life*: The relapser, once educated and if he properly understands what he is going through, will be able to recognize warning signs or problems that trigger the relapse. He can create a list of his own personal warning signs or reasons why. This way, he can do something about the triggers and prevent them from happening. For example, she may notice that when she does certain activities or eats certain foods, relapse is initiated. Living a balanced diet and life should be prioritized to experience pain-free                                                     existence.

# Chapter 7

# Understanding TMS

## What is TMS?

The condition is given the name Tension Myositis Syndrome (TMS) by Dr. John E. Sarno. It has also been called Tension Myoneural Syndrome and lately, the Mind-Body Syndrome. According to its descriptions, the condition is characterized by psyche-generated or psychogenic nerve and musculoskeletal symptoms, one of the most common being back pain.

Dr. Sarno, who has written about Tension Myositis Syndrome in four of his books, spoke of the condition being involved in other disorders that features pain as well. The protocol for TMS treatment includes writing about the patients' emotional issues, education about the condition, and resumption of their normal lifestyle, with or without supporting counseling sessions or psychotherapy. These treatments are found to be very effective for treatment of psychosomatic symptoms that results in chronic pain. Statistically, TMS treatments are also found to have outperformed other treatments targeting the same symptoms with a different approach than that forwarded by Dr. Sarno.

## Symptoms and Diagnosis

Tension myositis syndrome has always been associated with chronic back pains; but many more types and locations of the pain are found to have been caused by the condition.

TMS symptoms may include either individual experience or in a combination of the following:

- Pain
- Weakness
- Numbness
- Stiffness
- Tingling
- Dermatological disorder
- Gastrointestinal problems
- Repetitive-strain injury

Although occurring most frequently as localized back pains, tension myoneural syndrome can also manifest on other parts of the body. It may be on the wrists, arms, knees or neck. It has also been found that the symptoms have a tendency to move around the body. It is a significant indicator that if the symptoms move locations during treatment, that the pain is from TMS.

Sarno and Schechter have proposed a list of criterion for the diagnosis of TMS:

- *A History of Other Psychosomatic Disorders*

  Tension headaches, irritable bowel movement and other psychosomatic disorders experienced in the past may be an indication that an individual is suffering from tension myositis syndrome.

- *The Lack of a Definite Physical Cause for the Symptoms*

  A completed physical examination and other imaging studies would be able to rule out the influence of any other serious physical conditions. For example, the herniation on the spinal discs is usually blamed for pain and numbness in certain areas, even if the herniation location is not correlated with the location of the symptom.

- *Tender Points*

    Medical doctors often use tender points in certain key areas in the body to pinpoint the affliction and the cause of the symptoms. In 99% of TMS-diagnosed patients, eight tender points are often seen: two tender points in the lateral upper buttocks, two in the lumbar paraspinal muscles and two more points in the upper trapezius muscles.

It is highly recommended for patients who think they have TMS to visit a traditional medical doctor first. That is to be able to fully ascertain that the symptoms are not from any underlying physical disorders.

## Treatments

Treatment for tension myositis syndrome is a protocol that includes proper education about the patient's condition, writing and contemplation about their emotional issues and finally, a resumption of their normal lifestyle. For patients that are not responding that much to the regular treatment, additional support is given through counseling sessions and possibly, psychotherapy.

- *Education about TMS*

    This may take form in various modes of media. It may be through lectures, visitations or reference materials such as texts and audio content. The education would cover both physiological and psychological aspects of the disorder. This would allow their patients to learn that their physical condition is actually normal, and that any pain and disability they have is actually a result of deconditioning, fear of the recurrence of pain and experiencing the same injury again.

- *Writing about their Emotional Issues*

Specialists in tension myoneural syndrome attribute the disorder's symptoms to repressed emotions and fears. In such situations, the best solution is an awareness of these emotions. By facing the repressed fears head-on, individuals suffering from TMS symptoms defeat the repression through constant practice of meditation techniques and daily psychological processing.

With this in mind, the patients going through TMS treatment are given two writing assignments that they have to continuously repeat over a period of time. It is to list down all the issues that may contribute to their repressed emotions. These include their personality traits, the current pressures in their life, their childhood traumas and experiences, as well as issues of mortality and aging. This would generally include situations and experiences where the patient represses anger and other negative emotions, consciously or otherwise. Their next assignment is to write down in-depth essays about each of the items in their list. By writing longer on each item that they have identified, the patient is forced to look at the issues closely and possibly find resolution for them. Even if they don't do so, it would still be beneficial for the treatment. Here, the patient themselves come to have more insight regarding their own issues. It is found to be more therapeutic rather than someone else giving their own opinions on the said issues.

- *Resumption of the Patient's Normal Lifestyle*

There are two steps to this part of the patient's treatment. Firstly, all regular physical activity is resumed. The patients are recommended to become gradually active and slowly return to their normal life. They are also encouraged to get rid of habits previously obtained as safety behaviors meant to protect their "damaged" area – the location of the symptoms. The second part to this step is to discontinue treatments like physical therapy and spinal manipulation. As the patient is properly diagnosed with tension myositis syndrome, any physical treatment that were meant for disorders caused by other physical disorders will only reinforce the erroneous structural "root" of pain and other symptoms.

- *Meetings for Support and Counseling*

For patients who have problems responding to the previous steps of the treatment for TMS, additional support meetings may be arranged. There they may receive help with exploring their emotional issues; they can also review their education to get more clarification to further enhance their knowledge of their condition.

- *Recovery Program and Psychotherapy*

For the patients who do not make prompt recovery upon completion of the treatment, extensions or repetition of the treatment is coupled with six to ten sessions of psychotherapy. It is considered to be an option only for the few serious cases that show almost no response to the treatments, this method uses analytically-oriented dynamic psychotherapy.

There are also recovery programs available, packaged into audio and video sessions that are specially designed to cover the therapeutic concepts. The articles, segments and exercises are made to exemplify the healing process thus starting the treatment for the condition.

## Studies, Theory and Controversy

Tension myositis syndrome is a more controversial modality than pain disorder and psychogenic pain, both of which are now accepted diagnoses in the community of medicine. Multiple studies have already been made to attest the effectiveness of the treatments associated with TMS.

Researchers have stated that there is an advantage in the way that TMS treatments don't recommend medicine prescriptions and surgical procedures; it avoids the many risks. But since the disorder is relatively new, and the patients having been diagnosed and treated for it are still relatively low in number, any risk of the treatment is unknown.

The theory behind TMS, according to Dr. Sarno, is that the condition is initiated by unconscious emotional issues causing the symptoms, most particularly the manifestation of pain. It is suggested that, by using the autonomic nervous system, the unconscious mind decreases blood flow to certain areas of the body such as tendons, muscles and nerves that results to oxygen deprivation. This will then manifest as pain in the tissues affected. The most prominent characteristic to this condition is the migration of the pained area up and down the spine or from side to side. This movement implies that the pain may not be caused by any injury or physical deformity.

The theory then states that as a defense mechanism, the patient's mind uses the pain as a distraction from unconscious negative emotions and mental stress. This could be unconscious anxiety, anger and narcissistic rage. As the conscious mind is distracted by the pain, this type of psychological repression prevents the negative emotions from spilling out, keeping it tightly in the unconscious mind instead.

Dr. Sarno has always been a critic of conventional medicine diagnoses regarding back pain. As the usual treatments for them are rest, exercise, and physical therapy – with or without the surgery – they usually reinforce the emotional repression, and restrict the pain into the physical awareness.

The diagnosis and treatment for tension myoneural syndrome are not accepted to the majority of the medical community. But although mainstream medicine does not accept it, there are many notable doctors who do include TMS in the possible causes of localized pains and recommend TMS treatment for them.

The controversy of TMS as a theory and the effectiveness of its treatment reside in the fact that it hasn't been proven in a clinical trial that has been properly controlled. This quality is an inherent difficulty in conducting clinical trials for all psychosomatic illnesses such as TMS. Critics attribute its massive success rate into "placebo effect" and "regression to the mean" as there is only a small number of cases that are diagnosed and treated. It is also attributed to the fact that most cases of back pain resolve themselves within a few weeks. This is countered by TMS treatment doctors by responding that their successfully recovered patients are those who have approached and have been treated by them only after exhausting all other possibility of any underlying physical or psychological disorder in mainstream medicine. And that these people relied on them as a last resort. Indeed, it is highly recommended by TMS doctors to be completely sure that there are no underlying physical causes for their condition, with the proof subject to their evaluation.

## Other Important Notes about TMS

Here are some other suggestions with this book's very own commentaries that are from various resources that deal with tension myositis syndrome:

- *Your Own Inner Witness*

  In many TMS materials, experiences in the past where the individual experiences negative emotions can cause trouble and pain later on. Usually, people are able to express their emotions fluently as normal. And then after a period of time, they would just stop and move on from the issue; that is, even if their mind is still not ready for the recovery. This would result in a repressed emotion that will stay in the unconscious. When triggered or pressured, these will manifest into physical pain and other conditions like skin disorders and gastrointestinal anxiety to distract the mind away from emotional and psychological stress.

- *Nobody is Perfect*

One of the most common psychological stresses that causes tension myoneural syndrome is the daily demand for a person to work harder, to be good, to please everyone, to succeed; in short, to be perfect. The pain is made by the mind to distract the self from the rising anger of being unable to be so, and not wanting to answer to these demands. This conflict can be resolved by the realization of this issue, combined with self-acceptance and contentment exercises – counting what you have, opposed to focusing on what you don't, celebrating what you've achieved rather than looking back on what you failed upon – that will help ease the pressure you have placed on yourself.

- *Reflection is One of Your Best Weapons*

One of the major steps in the treatment of the mind-body syndrome is to write down your issues and contemplate on them. One has to practice reflection as often as they can for this to work. It is usually hard for individuals to reflect deeper and delve into their unconscious issues. That is because these are usually conglomerations of many factors that includes their entire emotional history, their personality traits, their current issues in life, as well as how they view the world and how they think the world views them. The key to reflection is to discard the fear of seeing something in yourself that you do not like. The more you shy away from the unpleasant facets of yourself, the more your unconscious will bury the important things away from your awareness.

- *Placebo Effectiveness*

Many who are aware that their pain has come from psychosomatic roots may have tried placebo treatments. Critics actually attribute the success of TMS treatments to the placebo effect. The only problem lies on the possibility of repeat episodes of the disorder after such a method. Time and time again, it has been proven that the human mind is a wonderful thing able to do such amazing feats. And this is the root of the placebo effect. Placebo treatments rely on the patient's complete belief that they are being treated, so their mind therefore, will treat the body accordingly. Just like how humans, by habit and conditioning, have learned to feel hungry at certain times in a day. That is, although humans can survive ingesting sustenance only once a day, or every few days for that matter, they have learned to "need" three full meals in daily. Although TMS treatment is not entirely in the placebo category, it does utilize the great power of the mind to heal itself.

- *Growing your Own Pain*

Once a certain negative emotion takes root in your unconscious, you naturally stack them up over time. The mind is a very organized being, no matter how chaotic you think your thought processes are. Human minds tend to categorize things and stack similar thoughts together. This naturally applies to the unconscious mind as well. This is the very reason why you can recall other instances that made you cry when you start crying. The mind links one memory with others that have the same emotional pull or significance. That is to say, unconscious anger will continue to build up as long as you are not aware of it enough to vent it. And soon, it will be causing unnecessary tension that will manifest into TMS pain and symptoms. One way to avoid this is to deal with an emotion as soon as they are formed. It may be awkward at first, but it will surely help in the long run. Get mad when you're angry, cry when you feel like doing so and vent all the bad things out whenever you can. If you can resolve the smaller issues just when they come into being, the faster you will be able to truly move on from them. That is, to avoid keeping them in, to be dealt in at a more "appropriate" time. There is no such thing, if you feel it now, deal with it now. It will save you from further self-incrimination in the future.

- *Awareness of your Habits and Behavioral Patterns*

Some people may react to stress by turning in to themselves. They tighten their face and head muscles which will definitely result in a headache later on. Others dilate or constrict blood vessels that limit the blood flow and therefore deprive certain body parts from much needed oxygen. Pain would then be experienced, including migraines and other localized pains because of this. The habits may not be observable easily, but with proper diagnosis and monitoring, these stress reactions can be removed by habitually practicing a conscious relaxation from the tension. Identifying when exactly that is may be difficult, since it would have been ingrained so deep into the person's habit that it would be indistinguishable from other involuntary body activity. For this, there are devices that can be requested to be used – called biofeedback – that will tell you when your body keeps on regressing into tension. A woman who had a case of temporo-mandibular disorder was found to have the habit of tensing her neck and jaws when she's stressed. Trying out the biofeedback device, the electronic box almost constantly lighted up, telling her that she's doing "it" again. After relaxation practice, which took some time getting used to, she's able to remove her habit and is now pain-free.

- *Overcoming Safety Behaviors, Awareness*

Usually when people experience pain, they tend to rely on deeply ingrained medical teachings on how to "take care" of one's body while it is "damaged". This usually involves avoiding certain physical activities that are deemed to be too strenuous and might have even caused the damage before. Because of this, lifestyles may be hindered and normal life is interrupted. It is as if time has come to a stagnant stop until the pain goes away, so that you can go back to what you were doing before. But the pain doesn't go; so you wait more, doing next to nothing. If you are diagnosed with TMS, you have to get rid of that habit of treating yourself as if you're breakable. The thought that you are fragile in your condition, and the fear that one wrong movement will cause pain, make up for a huge reinforcement to your stress. These in turn, will cause more pain.

- *Triggers*

Once you have identified your key issues that are the source of your TMS syndromes, you should also be able to see exactly what triggers reactions to these emotions. Subtle reminders from both the environment and your thought processes my trigger pain relapses. If you can pinpoint these triggers, you can analyze why exactly you are linking them to previously experienced issues. This way, you are processing more and more of the emotional impacts of your experiences. Awareness is one of the key features used in tension myositis syndrome treatment. The more you know, the more you are able to sort out the issues from within themselves. Doing so will make the inherent repression useless and the physical pain distraction to be unnecessary.

- *Understanding to Heal*

Healing psychosomatic disorders such as TMS basically requires a combination of understanding your condition, the reason why it came to be and a sort of constant self-reflection. Internal conflicts are usually the root of psychosomatic disorders. Resolving those conflict will ease up the pressure that the resulting stress has caused, leading into a gradual self-healing.

One of the things you have to understand is that there are a large number of people who are also experiencing the same things you are. That they are also suffering from the same pain you do even if it is in a different intensity in a different body part. You are not alone and you are not prohibited from asking help. Connecting with people who are going through the same things you are is a good way to slowly accept your condition. None of the treatments can ever help you if you do not accept that you are suffering from the condition in the first place. Many people have difficulties in doing so, preferring to blame it on a physical injury or disorder, on something that they can take a pill or have a surgery for. The fear of facing one's self and acknowledging that the problem is within you is one of the biggest hurdles that a TMS sufferer has to face. But it is not so much of a bother to those who have gone through almost all physical treatments, as they have already realized that the problem is not with their body but in their mind. That is why those who have gone through various physical therapies and such in the past respond more favorably to TMS treatments than those who have resorted to it earlier.

- *Personalities and Low Self-Esteem Causing Pain*

Certain personality traits like being a perfectionist or a pessimist can result to the manifestation of tension myositis syndrome. The compulsive, nearly obsessive preoccupation with perfecting everything and the fear of failure, as well as thoughts of things going wrong can put quite a strain on a person's psyche. The pressure can then be repressed through the unconscious mind by distracting the self with psychosomatic physical pains. And because these are personality traits that are formed over a person's lifetime, it is harder to identify and even more difficult to change.

Low self-esteem is also a leading cause of TMS symptoms. It causes a person to be very cautious in their every move and generally too careful with their dealings with others. As the pessimistic-version of the urge for perfection is amplified, the more the unconscious mind might be strained to the point of transferring the pressure into a physical distraction, as mentioned before.

- *Rage and Withholding Anger*

Withholding anger, most especially explosive rage, puts a massive pressure on the unconscious mind. Consciously swallowing your anger can be very destructive, turning your violent thoughts inward, causing stress for your emotions. Also, not letting anyone know of your emotional upheaval does not resolve the root. The rage would just simmer and be very sensitive. Flicking towards the boiling point over every little trigger-reminder you encounter.

Lately, this has seen many solutions. With the advent of internet and anonymous social media, one can freely express their anger, flinging it into the universe instead of keeping it in. Of course, there are still a lot of people who have made turning anger inwards a habit. For these people, they should have a way to vent their anger and frustration to ease the emotional stress that such feelings bring onto their own mind.

This could be in a form of a journal or diary, where the person can just write down everything that is going through their mind. There is actually a case where a teenage girl suffering from constant chest aches and "heavy feelings", has never been attributed to any existing physical cause. After discovering that she has a habit of not speaking at their school, she is made to keep a "Poison Notebook" where she writes down all the bad things she kept on thinking about other people. After a month of doing so, she returned to her sessions reporting the loss of her chest aches and a general decline in the "viciousness" of her thoughts. The counselor was presented her notebook and it was marked that, after a few weeks of endless notes dripping pure vitriol, her thought-notes have become less malign.

For other people, physical "violence" is the best way to vent anger. Hitting pillows, punching sandbags and such actions can help them fizzle out their rage. There is actually this one organization that has a "Rage Wall". People can come to their place filled with plates, cups, glasses, vases, pots and even appliances like old, unused TVs and radios. The visitors can then just keep on grabbing the items and throw them at the wall decorated with speech bubbles saying, "I hate you!" "Go fall in a ditch and die!" "Damn you!" and other angry lines that people can aim their plate – or cup, or TV – at. There is only one rule in the place. Don't hit anyone, just the walls.

- *Highly Sensitive People and those with Too Much Need for Attention*

These kinds of people generally think they are very fragile. And a deep-seated thought like that could make the notion a reality. These traits are usually a leftover characteristic from a previous experience that can date back to their childhood years. They tend to over-analyze things and overthink every little comment directed at them. This habit can create imaginary stress on a person's mind that can result in emotional pressures that are very real, leading up to a TMS-prone constitution.

- *Depression, Fatigue and Anxiety*

Depression, fatigue and anxiety can be very stressing to handle for the mind. Being unable to relax for long periods of time can hurt a person's unconscious mind. One of the traits common to these three, is the inability to share their condition with anyone. It could be because of situational

36

circumstances or a disinclination to do so. Because of the heightened stress on the psyche, coupled with the weakening of the physical, these can contribute to the appearance of TMS symptoms such as migraines and body pain.

- *Drugs and Pain*

Many psychosomatic disorders that feature pain as a symptom are wrongfully diagnosed as other physical illness. These people are then prescribed with pain medication. Now, since pain-reducing medicine target the actual area of the affliction – for example, the lower back – they are unable to ease the pain. Why? That is because the symptom is induced straight at the part of the brain dealing with the feeling of pain. And since the prescription does not help with the pain, the dosage or the medication strength is increased, with the same result. They end up desensitizing the body from the pain medication, rendering them ineffective at the instances that they are truly needed. Not only that, but you are also endangering the function of your organs that receive the stress of continuously ingesting the medication. The building up of the substances in your body may cause trouble in the near future.

- *Healing Yourself*

In all psychosomatic disorders such as tension myositis syndrome, self-healing is the most important facet of the treatment. Some people may prefer to let someone – usually their doctor – to boss them around, to tell them what to do and what not to do, what to eat, what they can't. This way the blame is on the physician when the treatment doesn't succeed. This should be changed. Even with conventional physical treatments, one should lord over themselves. This means accepting the healing and telling their body to recover. Without the will and determination to be healed, treatments would be just that – treatments – and not solutions.

37

- *Visualization and Setting Goals*

In connection to healing oneself, visualization and setting goals are important. You should have one big goal – to fully heal and return to normal, or an even better life – and some small milestones you will set for yourself. Visualizing a life where you are pain-less and is free to do whatever you want can help in cementing your determination to heal. This will also keep you up when the emotionally-taxing treatment brings you a bit down. By setting a final goal at the end of smaller goals, the big one feels easier. This is achieved by slowly traversing through the smaller goals one by one. Set a daily or weekly goal and visualize what you will be able to think and do by the end of that time period. Always give yourself some time to feel the celebration of your accomplishment for every milestone. Not only will it give you a needed break in your climb towards betterment, you will also feel more encouraged to go on and reach the final goal.

- *Communication*

Communication is very important in all treatments, most especially for psychosomatic conditions. Firstly, that should be with your doctor or counselor. Making regular updates with your progress can help them assess any need for adjustment and can also encourage you when you are hesitating in stepping onward. Communicating with your friends and family can provide immense amounts of support. Psychosomatic treatments can be very trying for relationships, but the best ones weather through by constant support and understanding. You'll come out of the experience together even closer and tighter than before. Also, communicating with other people suffering the same conditions as you do can be quite a help. With the internet and other forms of communication, it would be easy to get connected with these people. It is still quite a different kind of support to give and receive encouragements from people who are experiencing the same things as you do. The feeling of helping others out is also quite a good addition to your self-healing.

- *Mindful Meditation*

Many relaxation techniques and meditation exercises can be combined with an ongoing TMS treatment. By meditating, the patient can better explore their psyche and emotions as well as relaxing the body to let go of the involuntary tensions. These usually cause the pain and fatigue that are characteristic to psychosomatic disorders. Chronic pain sufferers tend to think "this will go on forever", "I'll never get better" or "I'm no good for anything anymore." By meditating on the positives and encouraging oneself, such hurdles are crossed and stresses are released, readying the mind and body for the healing to set in.

- *Laughter*

As always, laughter is still the best medicine. Induced feeling of happiness or even generally feeling good can do wonders for your condition. Doing fun things, watching funny movies and shows, or even just finding something to laugh at, helps you get over your negative emotions. Have fun with your friends and family. Enjoy hilarity wherever you can find them. Look into the brighter side of things. Soon enough, you'll be laughing at your previous worries like a wise man (or woman).

- *Comfort your Enemy*

In these treatments, your worst enemy is yourself. It is observed that people are generally more able to give advice and think of solutions for problems and anxieties of other people. So think of your own situations objectively. Comfort and give advice to yourself as if you're helping your best friend, or a close family. You are your greatest friend and your closest family after all; just as you are your worst enemy. It works both ways, you know. Of course, such an activity that requires clarity of thought and focus of your mind requires that you, yourself has identified what exactly is wrong. So dig in and help that pain-filled, trembling you inside that darkened interior of your heart.

- *Letting Go*

  There are root-causes for TMS that cannot be resolved either because they are entirely out of your control or because they are in the past and long gone. It is very painful to blame yourself for something that you have no control over. It has been one of the leading causes for TMS symptoms and are usually either self-imposed or are drilled into them all throughout a significant period of time. It could also be an experience long gone in the past that no one can do anything about anymore. In such cases, letting go would be the best option. One cannot totally forget memories, especially those that are heavy enough to cause impacts that affect you physically in the present. But they can be accepted, acknowledged and regarded as valuable stepping stones for the current you to reach where you are now. Don't endanger the future for something that happened in the past. Let them be your inspiration, your motivation to keep moving forward and up, instead of taking them with you like shackles that remind you of the pain. Don't live in the past, gradually move on into the present and be hopeful for your future.

These notes can be treated more like a points-to-ponder for your TMS education. This is an integral part of the treatment towards a pain-free lifestyle. Complete peace and contentment with your own body and life may be impossible, but striving towards it – without stressing yourself; never that, it's counterproductive – is a good course to follow.

# Conclusion

Thank you again for purchasing this book!

I hope this book was able to help you understand what pain is and how our body responds to painful stimulus. Furthermore, the objective of this book is to help you become aware of the negative effects pain can bring into your life and how you will be able to cope with it. There are several factors which can alleviate and aggravate pain and surely, you are already knowledgeable about those things. The next step is to apply this learning and share these helpful tips and information to other people, especially to those who are currently undergoing painful recovery.

Always remember that pain is only temporary. It goes away after the wound is healed. You have to accept that pain is a part of life and it is normal to be hurt sometimes. Do not succumb to the depressing stage of that painful experience. Pain is inevitable, but suffering is optional. Learn how to be strong and cope with pain accordingly. Do not suppress yourself. Share your pain with your loved ones because if pain is shared, it becomes more bearable. Never try to carry it all by yourself. After all, there really is no name for the pain.

Be hungry for the pain free life you deserve. Don't stop till you achieve relief from your symptoms. Dig deep to find the root causes and dig them out of your life. Keep persevering until you find the results you are looking for. Don't settle for status quo...you are worth much more than that. Your body is designed to be healthy and to live life to its fullest. Have hope for a future that is pain free.

In addition, please remember to check out our Facebook page in order to find other resources and upcoming promotions:

https://www.facebook.com/joypublishing

Thank you, from the bottom of my heart and I wish you the best.

With gratitude,

*Mia Soleil*

**Mia Soleil**

# Preview of "Fibromyalgia Book Guide" - How to Successfully Live with Fibromyalgia and Recipes for the Fibromyalgia Diet

# CHAPTER 1: DEALING WITH FIBROMYALGIA

Fibromyalgia is classified as a chronic disorder that is non-threatening. It is associated with a widespread pain in the musculoskeletal accompanied with mood, stress, fatigue, and sleep issues. Understand that fibromyalgia is not a disease, but a syndrome. It won't threaten your life, but the pain may become unbearable at any given time.

Most sufferers describe the condition as if they have persistent flu. The pain is all over the body and it has also been linked to anxiety, headaches, and depression. Although there is no proof that diet can indeed alleviate the symptoms of fibromyalgia, sufferers of the condition who chose to change their lifestyle and diet have seen significant improvement. If it worked for them, it will certainly do anyone suffering from the condition some good too, including you.

## The Pain is Not Just in Your Head

Because fibromyalgia is practically invisible, meaning X-rays or most lab tests do not and cannot give measurable findings regarding the condition, it does not mean that the pain you feel is just in your head. The pain is real and although it does not have any ability to inflict damage on the organs of your body or your joints, the relentless experience of being in pain can leave a significant influence in dealing with daily life.

The pain that comes with fibromyalgia can be so intense that some sufferers were once convinced that the pain they felt was only in their heads and there was no actual body pain: their brain just played tricks on them. The reason for such belief was due to the lack of evidence that such pain was possible since no X-rays or tests could corroborate the claim of the sufferers.

Currently, the medical community acknowledges the fact that the pain that is associated with having fibromyalgia is real. According to a research, it may have been caused by a glitch in the manner that the body perceives or senses the pain. The researchers believe that the condition intensifies the painful feelings by influencing the processing of pain signals in the brain.

The symptoms sometimes start after a major psychological stress, surgery, physical trauma, or infection. There are also cases where symptoms slowly accumulate within a certain period of time with unknown trigger.

## Risk Factors and Complications

Women are more likely to have fibromyalgia than men and it is also possible to develop it if someone in your family (a relative) has the condition too.

Several individuals who have fibromyalgia also experience having temporomandibular joint (TMJ) disorders, tension headaches, depression, anxiety, and irritable bowel syndrome (IBS).

There is no known cure for fibromyalgia, but there are available medications that can help alleviate the symptoms and let you go through the day without so much trouble. Good diet, exercise, stress-reduction procedures, and good amount of relaxation may also aid in alleviating the symptoms of fibromyalgia.

Individuals with lupus or rheumatoid arthritis and other rheumatic diseases are also more likely to have fibromyalgia.

The pain and lack of good sleep due to fibromyalgia can impede your ability to function properly at work or at home. The frustrations of handling the often misunderstood condition that sufferers feel can lead to health-related anxiety and depression.

It is best to take necessary measures and start practicing healthy lifestyle if you are someone who is at risk in developing the condition, already experiencing it, or has the condition already. Eating a well-balanced diet and avoiding certain foods, having a regular workout routine, and maintaining a stress free life can help a lot in keeping the condition under control.

## Symptoms of Fibromyalgia

The most typical symptom of fibromyalgia is a widespread pain (the sufferer experiences pain on both sides of the body, as well as above and below the waist) that could last for at least three months. There are cases wherein pain literally becomes a typical occurrence in the daily life of the victim. Although the sufferer should get used to the situation already, it can still affect the day to day existence of the affected person because the pain is real and not just in that person's head.

Sufferers of fibromyalgia often wake up in the morning feeling sluggish and tired although they have been sleeping for a long period of time. Sleep is often interrupted by pain, and several fibromyalgia victims have sleep disorders like apnea and restless legs syndrome.

There exists a symptom that is typically referred to as "fibro fog" which impairs the ability of the fibromyalgia patients to focus, concentrate on the work at hand, and pay attention.

Many individuals who suffer from fibromyalgia may also have constant headaches and cramps in the lower abdomen.

Women with fibromyalgia may experience more intense pain when they have the mentioned symptoms.

## Possible Causes of Fibromyalgia

Medical authorities are still baffled regarding the real culprits or causes of fibromyalgia, but they suspect that it involves several factors that come together to make the pain so intense.

It has been established that fibromyalgia may run in the family: certain genetic mutations may take place and make the sufferer more susceptible to the condition.

*Check out the rest of this book on Amazon*

Or go to: http://amzn.to/1eooSGX

# Check Out My Other Books

Below you'll find some of my other books that are popular on Amazon and Kindle as well. You can visit my author page on Amazon to see other work done by me. Alternatively, you can simply search for these titles on the Amazon website to find them.

.

**Eczema Treatment Guide: How to Live Pain Free with Natural Eczema Treatments and Eczema Diet Recipes**

**Fibromyalgia Book Guide: How to Successfully Live with Fibromyalgia and Recipes for the Fibromyalgia Diet**

If the links do not work, for whatever reason, you can simply search for these titles on the Amazon website to find them.

# One Last Thing...

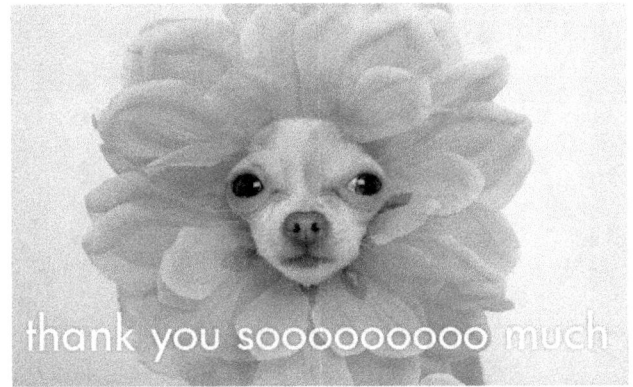

Source: Wikipedia

If you believe that this book is worth sharing, would you please take the time to let others know how it affected your life? If it turns out to make a difference in the lives of others, they will be forever grateful to you, as will I.

www.ingramcontent.com/pod-product-compliance
Lightning Source LLC
Chambersburg PA
CBHW070459290526
45790CB00003B/1018